This Bucket list belong to:

_____

_____

My Bucket List Goal _____
_____

Date _____ Location _____

Reason of doing this:
_____
_____
_____
_____

Actions we have to take:
_____
_____
_____
_____
_____
_____

My Experience:
_____
_____
_____
_____
_____

My Bucket List Goal ----- -----

Date ----- ----- Location ----- -----

Reason of doing this:

----- -----
----- -----
----- -----
----- -----

Actions we have to take:

----- -----
----- -----
----- -----
----- -----
----- -----

My Experience:

----- -----
----- -----
----- -----
----- -----

My Bucket List Goal ....

....

Date .... Location ....

Reason of doing this:

....

....

....

....

Actions we have to take:

....

....

....

....

....

....

My Experience:

....

....

....

....

....

My Bucket List Goal _____

_____

Date _____ Location _____

Reason of doing this:

_____

_____

_____

_____

Actions we have to take:

_____

_____

_____

_____

_____

_____

My Experience:

_____

_____

_____

_____

_____

_____

My Bucket List Goal _____
_____

Date _____   Location _____

Reason of doing this:
_____
_____
_____
_____

Actions we have to take:
_____
_____
_____
_____
_____
_____

My Experience:
_____
_____
_____
_____
_____

My Bucket List Goal _____

_____

Date _____ Location _____

Reason of doing this:

_____
_____
_____
_____

Actions we have to take:

_____
_____
_____
_____
_____
_____

My Experience:

_____
_____
_____
_____
_____

My Bucket List Goal _____

_____

Date _____ Location _____

Reason of doing this:

_____
_____
_____
_____

Actions we have to take:

_____
_____
_____
_____
_____
_____

My Experience:

_____
_____
_____
_____
_____

My Bucket List Goal _____

_____

Date _____   Location _____

Reason of doing this:

_____
_____
_____
_____

Actions we have to take:

_____
_____
_____
_____
_____
_____

My Experience:

_____
_____
_____
_____
_____

My Bucket List Goal

_____

_____

Date _____ Location _____

Reason of doing this:

_____

_____

_____

_____

Actions we have to take:

_____

_____

_____

_____

_____

_____

My Experience:

_____

_____

_____

_____

_____

_____

My Bucket List Goal _____

_____

Date _____ Location _____

Reason of doing this:

_____

_____

_____

_____

Actions we have to take:

_____

_____

_____

_____

_____

My Experience:

_____

_____

_____

_____

My Bucket List Goal

Date _____ Location _____

Reason of doing this:

_____

_____

_____

_____

Actions we have to take:

_____

_____

_____

_____

_____

_____

My Experience:

_____

_____

_____

_____

_____

My Bucket List Goal _____

_____

Date _____ Location _____

Reason of doing this:

_____
_____
_____
_____

Actions we have to take:

_____
_____
_____
_____
_____
_____

My Experience:

_____
_____
_____
_____
_____

My Bucket List Goal

Date _____ Location _____

Reason of doing this:

_____

_____

_____

_____

Actions we have to take:

_____

_____

_____

_____

_____

_____

My Experience:

_____

_____

_____

_____

_____

My Bucket List Goal _____

_____

Date _____ Location _____

Reason of doing this:

Actions we have to take:

My Experience:

My Bucket List Goal _____
_____

Date _____ Location _____

Reason of doing this:
_____
_____
_____
_____

Actions we have to take:
_____
_____
_____
_____
_____
_____

My Experience:
_____
_____
_____
_____
_____

My Bucket List Goal ....

....

Date .... Location ....

Reason of doing this:

....

....

....

....

Actions we have to take:

....

....

....

....

....

....

My Experience:

....

....

....

....

My Bucket List Goal _____

_____

Date _____ Location _____

Reason of doing this:

_____
_____
_____
_____

Actions we have to take:

_____
_____
_____
_____
_____
_____

My Experience:

_____
_____
_____
_____
_____

My Bucket List Goal ----------

Date ---------- Location ----------

Reason of doing this:

Actions we have to take:

My Experience:

My Bucket List Goal _____

_____

Date _____   Location _____

Reason of doing this:

_____

_____

_____

_____

Actions we have to take:

_____

_____

_____

_____

_____

_____

My Experience:

_____

_____

_____

_____

_____

My Bucket List Goal _____

_____

Date _____   Location _____

Reason of doing this:

_____

_____

_____

_____

Actions we have to take:

_____

_____

_____

_____

_____

My Experience:

_____

_____

_____

_____

_____

My Bucket List Goal ----- ----- -----

----- ----- ----- ----- ----- -----

Date ----- -----   Location ----- -----

Reason of doing this:

----- ----- ----- ----- ----- -----

----- ----- ----- ----- ----- -----

----- ----- ----- ----- ----- -----

----- ----- ----- ----- ----- -----

Actions we have to take:

----- ----- ----- ----- ----- -----

----- ----- ----- ----- ----- -----

----- ----- ----- ----- ----- -----

----- ----- ----- ----- ----- -----

----- ----- ----- ----- ----- -----

----- ----- ----- ----- ----- -----

My Experience:

----- ----- ----- ----- ----- -----

----- ----- ----- ----- ----- -----

----- ----- ----- ----- ----- -----

----- ----- ----- ----- ----- -----

----- ----- ----- ----- ----- -----

----- ----- ----- ----- ----- -----

My Bucket List Goal _____
_____

Date _____   Location _____

Reason of doing this:

_____
_____
_____
_____

Actions we have to take:

_____
_____
_____
_____
_____
_____

My Experience:

_____
_____
_____
_____

My Bucket List Goal

_____

_____

Date _____ Location _____

Reason of doing this:

Actions we have to take:

My Experience:

My Bucket List Goal _____

Date _____ Location _____

Reason of doing this:

_____
_____
_____
_____

Actions we have to take:

_____
_____
_____
_____
_____

My Experience:

_____
_____
_____
_____
_____

My Bucket List Goal _____

_____

Date _____ Location _____

Reason of doing this:

_____
_____
_____
_____

Actions we have to take:

_____
_____
_____
_____
_____
_____

My Experience:

_____
_____
_____
_____
_____

My Bucket List Goal _____

Date _____ Location _____

Reason of doing this:

_____
_____
_____
_____

Actions we have to take:

_____
_____
_____
_____
_____

My Experience:

_____
_____
_____
_____

My Bucket List Goal _____

_____

Date _____ Location _____

Reason of doing this:

_____
_____
_____
_____

Actions we have to take:

_____
_____
_____
_____
_____
_____

My Experience:

_____
_____
_____
_____
_____

My Bucket List Goal _____

_____

Date _____ Location _____

Reason of doing this:

_____
_____
_____
_____

Actions we have to take:

_____
_____
_____
_____
_____

My Experience:

_____
_____
_____
_____
_____

My Bucket List Goal _____

_____

Date _____ Location _____

Reason of doing this:

_____

_____

_____

_____

Actions we have to take:

_____

_____

_____

_____

_____

_____

My Experience:

_____

_____

_____

_____

_____

My Bucket List Goal _____

_____

Date _____ Location _____

Reason of doing this:

_____
_____
_____
_____

Actions we have to take:

_____
_____
_____
_____
_____
_____

My Experience:

_____
_____
_____
_____
_____

My Bucket List Goal

_____

_____

Date _____ Location _____

Reason of doing this:

_____

_____

_____

_____

Actions we have to take:

_____

_____

_____

_____

_____

My Experience:

_____

_____

_____

_____

My Bucket List Goal _____

_____

Date _____ Location _____

Reason of doing this:

_____
_____
_____
_____

Actions we have to take:

_____
_____
_____
_____
_____
_____

My Experience:

_____
_____
_____
_____
_____

My Bucket List Goal _____

_____

Date _____ Location _____

Reason of doing this:

_____

_____

_____

_____

Actions we have to take:

_____

_____

_____

_____

_____

_____

My Experience:

_____

_____

_____

_____

_____

My Bucket List Goal

_____

_____

Date _____ Location _____

Reason of doing this:

_____

_____

_____

_____

Actions we have to take:

_____

_____

_____

_____

_____

My Experience:

_____

_____

_____

_____

My Bucket List Goal ....

....

Date .... Location ....

Reason of doing this:

....

....

....

....

Actions we have to take:

....

....

....

....

....

....

My Experience:

....

....

....

....

....

My Bucket List Goal _____

_____

Date _____ Location _____

Reason of doing this:

Actions we have to take:

My Experience:

My Bucket List Goal _____

_____

Date _____ Location _____

Reason of doing this:

_____

_____

_____

_____

Actions we have to take:

_____

_____

_____

_____

_____

_____

My Experience:

_____

_____

_____

_____

_____

My Bucket List Goal _____

_____

Date _____ Location _____

Reason of doing this:

_____
_____
_____
_____

Actions we have to take:

_____
_____
_____
_____
_____

My Experience:

_____
_____
_____
_____

My Bucket List Goal _____

_____

Date _____ Location _____

Reason of doing this:

_____

_____

_____

_____

Actions we have to take:

_____

_____

_____

_____

_____

_____

My Experience:

_____

_____

_____

_____

_____

My Bucket List Goal _
_ _

Date _ _ _ _ _ _ _ _ _ _ _ Location _ _ _ _ _ _ _ _ _ _ _ _ _

Reason of doing this:
_ _
_ _
_ _
_ _

Actions we have to take:
_ _
_ _
_ _
_ _
_ _

My Experience:
_ _
_ _
_ _
_ _

My Bucket List Goal _____

_____

Date _____ Location _____

Reason of doing this:

_____

_____

_____

_____

Actions we have to take:

_____

_____

_____

_____

_____

_____

My Experience:

_____

_____

_____

_____

_____

My Bucket List Goal _

_ _

Date _ _ _ _ _ _ _ _ _ _ _ _   Location _ _ _ _ _ _ _ _ _ _ _ _ _

Reason of doing this:

_ _

_ _

_ _

_ _

Actions we have to take:

_ _

_ _

_ _

_ _

_ _

My Experience:

_ _

_ _

_ _

_ _

My Bucket List Goal _____

_____

Date _____ Location _____

Reason of doing this:

_____

_____

_____

_____

Actions we have to take:

_____

_____

_____

_____

_____

My Experience:

_____

_____

_____

_____

_____

My Bucket List Goal _____

_____

Date _____ Location _____

Reason of doing this:

_____

_____

_____

_____

Actions we have to take:

_____

_____

_____

_____

_____

_____

My Experience:

_____

_____

_____

_____

_____

My Bucket List Goal

_____

_____

Date _____ Location _____

Reason of doing this:

_____
_____
_____
_____

Actions we have to take:

_____
_____
_____
_____
_____
_____

My Experience:

_____
_____
_____
_____
_____

My Bucket List Goal _____

_____

Date _____ Location _____

Reason of doing this:

_____

_____

_____

_____

Actions we have to take:

_____

_____

_____

_____

_____

My Experience:

_____

_____

_____

_____

My Bucket List Goal _____

_____

Date _____ Location _____

Reason of doing this:

_____

_____

_____

_____

Actions we have to take:

_____

_____

_____

_____

_____

_____

My Experience:

_____

_____

_____

_____

_____

_____

My Bucket List Goal _____

_____

Date _____ Location _____

Reason of doing this:

_____

_____

_____

_____

Actions we have to take:

_____

_____

_____

_____

_____

_____

My Experience:

_____

_____

_____

_____

_____

My Bucket List Goal ....
....

Date .... Location ....

Reason of doing this:
....
....
....
....

Actions we have to take:
....
....
....
....
....
....

My Experience:
....
....
....
....
....

My Bucket List Goal ----- ----- -----
----- ----- ----- ----- -----

Date ----- ----- ----- Location ----- ----- -----

Reason of doing this:

----- ----- ----- ----- -----
----- ----- ----- ----- -----
----- ----- ----- ----- -----
----- ----- ----- ----- -----

Actions we have to take:

----- ----- ----- ----- -----
----- ----- ----- ----- -----
----- ----- ----- ----- -----
----- ----- ----- ----- -----
----- ----- ----- ----- -----
----- ----- ----- ----- -----

My Experience:

----- ----- ----- ----- -----
----- ----- ----- ----- -----
----- ----- ----- ----- -----
----- ----- ----- ----- -----

My Bucket List Goal _____

_____

Date _____ Location _____

Reason of doing this:

_____
_____
_____
_____

Actions we have to take:

_____
_____
_____
_____
_____
_____

My Experience:

_____
_____
_____
_____
_____
_____

My Bucket List Goal _____
_____

Date _____ Location _____

Reason of doing this:
_____
_____
_____
_____

Actions we have to take:
_____
_____
_____
_____
_____
_____

My Experience:
_____
_____
_____
_____

My Bucket List Goal _____

_____

Date _____ Location _____

Reason of doing this:

_____

_____

_____

_____

Actions we have to take:

_____

_____

_____

_____

_____

_____

My Experience:

_____

_____

_____

_____

_____

My Bucket List Goal _____

_____

Date _____ Location _____

Reason of doing this:

_____

_____

_____

_____

Actions we have to take:

_____

_____

_____

_____

_____

My Experience:

_____

_____

_____

_____

_____

My Bucket List Goal _____

_____

Date _____ Location _____

Reason of doing this:

Actions we have to take:

My Experience:

My Bucket List Goal _____

_____

Date _____ Location _____

Reason of doing this:

_____
_____
_____
_____

Actions we have to take:

_____
_____
_____
_____
_____
_____

My Experience:

_____
_____
_____
_____
_____

My Bucket List Goal

_____

_____

Date _____ Location _____

Reason of doing this:

_____

_____

_____

_____

Actions we have to take:

_____

_____

_____

_____

_____

_____

My Experience:

_____

_____

_____

_____

_____

My Bucket List Goal _____

_____

Date _____ Location _____

Reason of doing this:

_____
_____
_____
_____

Actions we have to take:

_____
_____
_____
_____
_____

My Experience:

_____
_____
_____
_____

My Bucket List Goal _____

_____

Date _____ Location _____

Reason of doing this:

_____

_____

_____

_____

Actions we have to take:

_____

_____

_____

_____

_____

My Experience:

_____

_____

_____

_____

_____

My Bucket List Goal _____

_____

Date _____ Location _____

Reason of doing this:

_____
_____
_____
_____

Actions we have to take:

_____
_____
_____
_____
_____

My Experience:

_____
_____
_____
_____

My Bucket List Goal _____

_____

Date _____ Location _____

Reason of doing this:

_____

_____

_____

_____

Actions we have to take:

_____

_____

_____

_____

_____

My Experience:

_____

_____

_____

_____

_____

My Bucket List Goal ....

....

Date .... Location ....

Reason of doing this:

....

....

....

....

Actions we have to take:

....

....

....

....

....

My Experience:

....

....

....

....

....

My Bucket List Goal ....

....

Date .... Location ....

Reason of doing this:

....
....
....
....

Actions we have to take:

....
....
....
....
....
....

My Experience:

....
....
....
....
....

My Bucket List Goal

Date _____ Location _____

Reason of doing this:

_____
_____
_____
_____

Actions we have to take:

_____
_____
_____
_____
_____

My Experience:

_____
_____
_____
_____

My Bucket List Goal

Date _____ Location _____

Reason of doing this:

_____
_____
_____
_____

Actions we have to take:

_____
_____
_____
_____
_____
_____

My Experience:

_____
_____
_____
_____
_____

My Bucket List Goal _____

_____

Date _____ Location _____

Reason of doing this:

_____
_____
_____
_____

Actions we have to take:

_____
_____
_____
_____
_____

My Experience:

_____
_____
_____
_____

My Bucket List Goal

Date _____ Location _____

Reason of doing this:

_____

_____

_____

_____

Actions we have to take:

_____

_____

_____

_____

_____

_____

My Experience:

_____

_____

_____

_____

_____

My Bucket List Goal

Date _____ Location _____

Reason of doing this:
_____
_____
_____
_____

Actions we have to take:
_____
_____
_____
_____
_____

My Experience:
_____
_____
_____
_____
_____

My Bucket List Goal

Date _____ Location _____

Reason of doing this:

_____

_____

_____

_____

Actions we have to take:

_____

_____

_____

_____

_____

_____

My Experience:

_____

_____

_____

_____

_____

_____

My Bucket List Goal _____

_____

Date _____ Location _____

Reason of doing this:

_____

_____

_____

_____

Actions we have to take:

_____

_____

_____

_____

_____

_____

My Experience:

_____

_____

_____

_____

My Bucket List Goal _____

_____

Date _____ Location _____

Reason of doing this:

_____

_____

_____

_____

Actions we have to take:

_____

_____

_____

_____

_____

_____

My Experience:

_____

_____

_____

_____

_____

My Bucket List Goal _____
_____

Date _____ Location _____

Reason of doing this:
_____
_____
_____
_____

Actions we have to take:
_____
_____
_____
_____
_____

My Experience:
_____
_____
_____
_____
_____

My Bucket List Goal ....

....

Date .... Location ....

Reason of doing this:

....

....

....

....

Actions we have to take:

....

....

....

....

....

....

My Experience:

....

....

....

....

....

....

My Bucket List Goal _____ _____ _____

_____ _____ _____ _____ _____

Date _____ _____ Location _____ _____

Reason of doing this:

_____ _____ _____ _____ _____
_____ _____ _____ _____ _____
_____ _____ _____ _____ _____
_____ _____ _____ _____ _____

Actions we have to take:

_____ _____ _____ _____ _____
_____ _____ _____ _____ _____
_____ _____ _____ _____ _____
_____ _____ _____ _____ _____
_____ _____ _____ _____ _____

My Experience:

_____ _____ _____ _____ _____
_____ _____ _____ _____ _____
_____ _____ _____ _____ _____
_____ _____ _____ _____ _____
_____ _____ _____ _____ _____

My Bucket List Goal _____

_____

Date _____ Location _____

Reason of doing this:

_____

_____

_____

_____

Actions we have to take:

_____

_____

_____

_____

_____

_____

My Experience:

_____

_____

_____

_____

_____

_____

My Bucket List Goal _____

_____

Date _____ Location _____

Reason of doing this:

_____
_____
_____
_____

Actions we have to take:

_____
_____
_____
_____
_____

My Experience:

_____
_____
_____
_____
_____

My Bucket List Goal _____

_____

Date _____ Location _____

Reason of doing this:

_____

_____

_____

_____

Actions we have to take:

_____

_____

_____

_____

_____

My Experience:

_____

_____

_____

_____

_____

My Bucket List Goal _____

_____

Date _____ Location _____

Reason of doing this:

_____
_____
_____
_____

Actions we have to take:

_____
_____
_____
_____
_____
_____

My Experience:

_____
_____
_____
_____

My Bucket List Goal

Date _____ Location _____

Reason of doing this:

- -

- -

- -

- -

Actions we have to take:

- -

- -

- -

- -

- -

- -

My Experience:

- -

- -

- -

- -

- -

My Bucket List Goal _____

_____

Date _____ Location _____

Reason of doing this:

_____

_____

_____

_____

Actions we have to take:

_____

_____

_____

_____

_____

_____

My Experience:

_____

_____

_____

_____

_____

My Bucket List Goal _____

_____

Date _____ Location _____

Reason of doing this:

_____

_____

_____

_____

Actions we have to take:

_____

_____

_____

_____

_____

_____

My Experience:

_____

_____

_____

_____

_____

My Bucket List Goal _____

_____

Date _____   Location _____

Reason of doing this:

_____
_____
_____
_____

Actions we have to take:

_____
_____
_____
_____
_____
_____

My Experience:

_____
_____
_____
_____
_____

My Bucket List Goal ....

Date .... Location ....

Reason of doing this:

....
....
....
....

Actions we have to take:

....
....
....
....
....
....

My Experience:

....
....
....
....
....
....

My Bucket List Goal ----------------------------

Date ------------------- Location --------------------

Reason of doing this:

Actions we have to take:

My Experience:

My Bucket List Goal _____

_____

Date _____ Location _____

Reason of doing this:

_____

_____

_____

_____

Actions we have to take:

_____

_____

_____

_____

_____

_____

My Experience:

_____

_____

_____

_____

_____

My Bucket List Goal ....
....

Date .... Location ....

Reason of doing this:
....
....
....
....

Actions we have to take:
....
....
....
....
....

My Experience:
....
....
....
....

My Bucket List Goal _____

_____

Date _____ Location _____

Reason of doing this:

_____

_____

_____

_____

Actions we have to take:

_____

_____

_____

_____

_____

_____

My Experience:

_____

_____

_____

_____

_____

My Bucket List Goal ⁣ ⁣

⁣

Date ⁣ ⁣ Location ⁣ ⁣

Reason of doing this:

⁣

⁣

⁣

⁣

Actions we have to take:

⁣

⁣

⁣

⁣

⁣

My Experience:

⁣

⁣

⁣

⁣

My Bucket List Goal _____

_____

Date _____ Location _____

Reason of doing this:

Actions we have to take:

My Experience:

My Bucket List Goal _____

_____

Date _____ Location _____

Reason of doing this:

Actions we have to take:

My Experience:

My Bucket List Goal

Date _____ Location _____

Reason of doing this:

_____

_____

_____

_____

Actions we have to take:

_____

_____

_____

_____

_____

_____

My Experience:

_____

_____

_____

_____

_____

My Bucket List Goal ----------------------------------

Date ---------------- Location -------------------------

Reason of doing this:

Actions we have to take:

My Experience:

My Bucket List Goal _____

_____

Date _____ Location _____

Reason of doing this:

_____

_____

_____

_____

Actions we have to take:

_____

_____

_____

_____

_____

_____

My Experience:

_____

_____

_____

_____

_____

My Bucket List Goal _____

Date _____   Location _____

Reason of doing this:

_____

_____

_____

_____

Actions we have to take:

_____

_____

_____

_____

_____

_____

My Experience:

_____

_____

_____

_____

My Bucket List Goal _____

_____

Date _____ Location _____

Reason of doing this:

- -

- -

- -

- -

Actions we have to take:

- -

- -

- -

- -

- -

- -

My Experience:

- -

- -

- -

- -

- -

My Bucket List Goal _____

_____

Date _____   Location _____

Reason of doing this:

_____

_____

_____

_____

Actions we have to take:

_____

_____

_____

_____

_____

_____

My Experience:

_____

_____

_____

_____

_____

My Bucket List Goal _____
_____

Date _____   Location _____

Reason of doing this:
_____
_____
_____
_____

Actions we have to take:
_____
_____
_____
_____
_____
_____

My Experience:
_____
_____
_____
_____
_____

My Bucket List Goal _____

_____

Date _____ Location _____

Reason of doing this:

_____

_____

_____

_____

Actions we have to take:

_____

_____

_____

_____

_____

_____

My Experience:

_____

_____

_____

_____

_____

My Bucket List Goal _____

_____

Date _____   Location _____

Reason of doing this:

_____

_____

_____

_____

Actions we have to take:

_____

_____

_____

_____

_____

_____

My Experience:

_____

_____

_____

_____

_____

My Bucket List Goal ....

....

Date .... Location ....

Reason of doing this:

....

....

....

....

Actions we have to take:

....

....

....

....

....

My Experience:

....

....

....

....

....

My Bucket List Goal _____

_____

Date _____ Location _____

Reason of doing this:

_____

_____

_____

_____

Actions we have to take:

_____

_____

_____

_____

_____

My Experience:

_____

_____

_____

_____

_____

My Bucket List Goal _____

_____

Date _____ Location _____

Reason of doing this:

_____

_____

_____

_____

Actions we have to take:

_____

_____

_____

_____

_____

_____

My Experience:

_____

_____

_____

_____

My Bucket List Goal ----------------------------------

Date - - - - - - - - - -   Location - - - - - - - - - -

Reason of doing this:

- -

- -

- -

- -

Actions we have to take:

- -

- -

- -

- -

- -

- -

My Experience:

- -

- -

- -

- -

- -

My Bucket List Goal _____
_____

Date _____ Location _____

Reason of doing this:
_____
_____
_____
_____

Actions we have to take:
_____
_____
_____
_____
_____
_____

My Experience:
_____
_____
_____
_____

My Bucket List Goal _____

_____

Date _____ Location _____

Reason of doing this:

_____

_____

_____

_____

Actions we have to take:

_____

_____

_____

_____

_____

_____

My Experience:

_____

_____

_____

_____

_____

My Bucket List Goal _____

_____

Date _____ Location _____

Reason of doing this:

_____

_____

_____

_____

Actions we have to take:

_____

_____

_____

_____

_____

_____

My Experience:

_____

_____

_____

_____

_____

My Bucket List Goal _____

_____

Date _____ Location _____

Reason of doing this:

_____

_____

_____

_____

Actions we have to take:

_____

_____

_____

_____

_____

_____

My Experience:

_____

_____

_____

_____

_____

My Bucket List Goal _____

_____

Date _____ Location _____

Reason of doing this:

Actions we have to take:

My Experience:

www.ingramcontent.com/pod-product-compliance
Lightning Source LLC
Chambersburg PA
CBHW020542220526
45463CB00006B/2161